The Secret of Body, Soul and Mind

Wolfgang Rietig

The Secret

of

Body, Soul and Mind

Other published works by the author W. Rietig:

"Phenomenon" Sudden Infant Death Syndrome – Finally Understood.
With therapy information for the adult

Healthy or exhausted?
Holistic therapy/Naturopathy
Pain-Heart-Circulation-Cancer

Living a longer active life!
Deacidifying-Cleansing-Detoxing
Cancer-Cancer prophylaxis

© 2010 Wolfgang Rietig
Cover design, layout, publishing and production:
Books on Demand GmbH, Norderstedt
ISBN 978-3-8391-9234-4

Elucidations whose contents do not appear to be known represent the views and experiences of the author.
The medical section is directed at the expectations of inner circles of experts.

Contents

The mysterious thoughts

Body – Soul and Mind!?
A lot has been written about the mind and soul. However, quite surprisingly, not a lot about the body and the functions and processes of its organs and their processes.
Our thoughts are still free and uncontrollable. You can develop best without rush, stress and, in particular, noise.
Peace and quiet is what we need most to achieve this. This, however, does not start with total silence but at a level below 40 decibel which applies, in particular, to the nightly sleeping time. Even people who can sleep in noisy surroundings take the detriments to health over into the waking hours the next day. Metabolic disorders, lowered resistance, cardiac problems, thyroid disorders and many other things all the way to cancer can be the result. Relaxation and listening to our body lets the mind and soul oscillate in a pleasant manner. Women all up live more perceptively. That is why they also experience negative vibes, no matter what their cause, with more psychological impact than men. The vastness which is perceived in silence gives us an indication of one's own boundlessness of the trip through eternity. If we are instilled with a good mind, our thoughts oscillate in a divine order corresponding with wellbeing. After all, the power of positive thoughts results not least from physical wellbeing. A healthy mind will not feel well in an ill body.
The body can be affected by a mental illness. In this case, the function of the subconsciousness, which is involved in metabolic processes, is irritated. Thoughts therefore come and go according to how we feel.
Our thoughts in their flow may end or loose themselves one day in our "being". In the silence we can then gather the strength which lets our mind and soul oscillate pleasantly. Let us treasure the silence of our thoughts as God's gift. Light, rhythmic alternating stress

between body, soul and mind has a beneficial effect. By contrast, constant stress damages all organ systems in an unpleasant manner. Countless bio-chemical reactions take place in just one second in each cell of the body. If these processes are impaired, the organism falls ill. The strength and intensity of our ability to believe depends on the overall physical health. Independent of the relationship which we are trying to have or maintain, the basic factor is which depth do we want in it.

The mysterious soul

At all times mankind has dealt with the question whether there is a soul. A Greek[1] born in 583 B.C, spoke about his viewpoint on the transmigration of souls in public, a view which was contrary to the then prevailing opinion.

Aristotle, who expanded the teachings of earlier philosophers, in particular Plato's, looked at the soul as a form principle of everything that lives.

The soul is an immortal energy formation and relates to the eternal existance.

It is assumed that the soul incarnates into the developing organism long before its birth. Emotional components such as happiness, love, sadness, disappointment and the blows of fate influence the soul according to their respective intensity. The emotions are perceived via the conscious and manifest themselves in the most varied forms.

Many people deny the existence of a soul. They simply do not believe in it and ignore the law of polarity, respectively opposites.

So many things are opposites, for example sun and moon, water and fire, cold and heat and so on. Electrical current cannot flow when there is no plus or minus, that is, the polar opposite. Current is invisible as are radio waves. If we turn the television on, we can see the visible image which could not exist without the invisible current. It follows that the visible body must have the invisible soul as polar opposite.

Since primeval times, mankind has been asking the question, what is the soul, respectively what does it look like. The author has also asked himself this question many times and has come to the following opinion: the soul is an invisible <u>energy formation</u>, consisting of cosmic radiation with specific oscillation character. An oscillation originates in the atom, where frequency means "oscillation per second". Our alternating current has a frequency of 50 Hertz and therefore oscillates

50 times per second. The soul is correlated to the mind and body, however it is an energy formation for itself with infinite knowledge in its energy spectrum, to which it owes its immortality. Every soul is unique. Who we are, how we are, what we are, is imprinted in it. The very own character of mankind is captured in it. The soul reacts to each deviation from this plan, to each disruption of this plan.

The soul is timeless. Just like the present, the past and the future are a large circle, where there is no beginning and no end. Time is an illusion created by mankind.

The soul appears again and again in various elucidations including proverbs. In the opinion of philosophers, the soul can leave[2] the body temporarily, something which can also happen during sleep. It would be in the position to stay in the present after the death of a person, or to travel to the invisible world in the hereafter. According to the doctrine of reincarnation the soul enters another body after death. If the soul leaves the body, it is no longer possible for the mind to remain in the body as one energy formation is dependent on the other. With each reincarnation, the soul has the opportunity to develop further, perhaps also the opportunity to work off, respectively solve mistakes from a past life. The events and skills developed by the soul in this life will manifest themselves as talents in the next life, similar to the passing on of genetic information across generations. But also fateful events and the consequences therefrom will still rise to the surface of the unconsciousness as sensations.

The meaning of life could therefore be further development of the soul. The longer we live, the more our soul can develop.

The belief that the soul can also be re-incarnated into an animal is widespread. The preferred host body is that of birds. According to the teachings of Hinduism, there is no difference between the souls of mankind and the souls of animals (holy cows).

All matter will be dissolved at some stage. It can therefore be assumed that a person whose soul is too extremely tied to money, will, at some stage cease to exist once the material or tangible is liquidated. Mankind looses its being.

The soul in its entity can be looked at as the biggest archive of information when it comes to storage and retentiveness. If a person is socially minded, helpful towards his neighbour, one speaks of a good soul.

It is not clear where in the body the soul could reside. A possible place would be, in the author's opinion, the region of the solar plexus (centre of feeling), from which it radiates to all parts of the body.

A rich man left a special legacy in Great Britain. The person who could prove the existence of the soul would be given 1 million pounds. Perhaps this will be possible one day, when quantum physics has developed further.

Classic homeopathy with its high-potencies could indicate the way. A high-potency of, for example, D500 (500 multiplied 10-times with itself) no longer contains anything of the original substance. The information increases in the manner in which the substance is diluted. One could here speak of sub-atomic energy. A few drops per year could put processes into action which would lead to the healing or removal of a symptom, respectively of an illness. It can be assumed that this process runs via the soul and acts on the organ systems. The processes must run in a similar way in animals, because healing processes turn up which the animal simply cannot imagine. The argument of the placebo effect should therefore be invalidated. We can assume that a homeopathic high-potency with its oscillations will combine with the oscillations of the soul and therefore the healing effect of the soul on the body with which it is associated, will take place. The soul acts from the inside to the outside.

The soul has a memory similar to a USB stick for a computer, where you can store a lot of information. Reports continuously state that one's whole life seems to flash past like a movie at high speed at the end, respectively while passing away. The soul knows all our difficulties and stress which we are exposed to. If we feel physically well, it influences our psychological wellbeing. This again has a favourable influence on the soul so that this can oscillate in a eutonic fashion. It is therefore definitely worthwhile strengthening the body as much as possible via holistic and naturopathic influences (described in more detail in Rietig, Wolfgang, Healthy or exhausted? **Holistic therapy/ Naturopathy Pain-Heart-Circulation-Cancer**").

If a person fells physically well, it is easier for him or her to think positively, something which brightness the psyche and strengthens the soul. The psyche, however, is not the soul as is often erroneously assumed. The psyche results from the performances of brain functions. It is the result of physical wellbeing and is in correlation with the oscillations of the soul. When this eutonic state predominates, it is easier to deal with the blows life deals out.

If the formation of carrier agents in the brain cells is disrupted because the body is flooded with toxins, it is inevitable that the transmission of nerve impulses from one cell to the other is also disrupted. The result is fear, depression and aggressiveness. This then leads to dysfunctions of the soul. Attempting to remove the fear and/or other symptoms will only work when the metabolism in the cells reverts back to a normal direction. Naturopathy has various homeopathic agents available to change these symptoms. Detoxing is essential because when the body is detoxed it also means relief for the soul because the symptoms burdening the soul are reduced. The excessive pursuit of possessions resulting from the conscious inevitably leads to an unhealthy emptiness, respectively paraesthesia in the soul. If we foster conscious thought in the direction of perceiving and observing positive coherences, we will be making a big step towards a good frame of mind.

Psychic wellbeing also depends very much on the vegetative nervous system. It consists of the stimulating part, the sympathetic nervous system and the inhibiting, sedating part, the parasympathetic nervous system, respectively the vagus (10th cranial nerve). It works autonomously and is independent of will. The sympathetic and para-sympathetic trunk should be in balance so that emotional wellbeing results.

This is seriously impaired when one of the vegetative parts is weakened through intoxication. Balance changes and environmental stress can no longer be compensated. We feel overwhelmed and can no longer cope with the slightest challenge. Lots of activity in the fresh air combined with periods of rest, a vitamin and mineral rich diet and plenty of vegetables have a strengthening effect on the vegetative system and therefore the psyche. Stimulants like coffee or tobacco should be avoided, as should too much alcohol because it acidifies the organism. A daily quantity of water of approx. 2-2.5 l as vehicle for excreting the toxins in the body is an absolute must!

For every creature, photo-metabolism with its corresponding effect on the organ systems and physiological processes in the body should also not be forgotten. Light contains different colours in a spectrum which also have an effect on the psyche. The oscillations, respectively frequencies of light coming from the sun are invisible. Once it enters earth's atmosphere it meets air molecules and becomes visible in the blue colouration. In contrast, the lunar sky is black as the beams of light only become visible when they hit the surface of the moon. If light is missing on cloudy, rainy days, a gloomy mood settles in which shrouds the mind and soul. In contrast, mood and energy levels improve when the sun shines. A lack of sunlight can also lead to, for example, cravings for chocolates and sweets. A lack of light can also effect tiredness, sleep disruptions and hyper-nervousness. It may be assumed that a lack of light not only stresses the body and psyche but also affects emotional feelings. Vicious behaviour and injustice from the world around us can damage a soul.

Permanent emotional or psychogenic damage often results in children whose parents neglect their parental custodial duties and who do not take care of the child properly. The soul of the child withers. It becomes aggressive, displays behavioural problems, turns violent or falls into a depression. It is worse still when an unsupervised child falls into the hands of a molester. The child suffers intense agonies before it is killed emotionally and/or physically.

If we move around a lot in the fresh air, we release hormones which also contribute towards psychic wellbeing and the emotions turn towards a good direction.

How each person develops, whether in a positive or negative direction, lies in their own hands due to their decision-making powers. If a person decides in favour of the positive he or she is rewarded with emotional wellbeing.

However, the increase of disasters shows us clearly that mankind does not live in harmony with nature, instead his behaviour is destructive to the highest degree. Water-ground-air have already reached a high degree of toxicity and irritate people's behaviour patterns.

It is generally assumed that there is a world soul. If one imagines the earth as visible polar opposite then, according to the law of polarity, there should inevitably be this invisible world soul. The ecologic destruction of the earth automatically attracts changes in the oscillation range. These changed oscillation frequencies then disrupt the oscillation character of the invisible soul energy which spans the earth. The denaturation of ground, water, air, nature, the emergence of the ozone hole through CFC and the electro-smog have long since influenced earth's oscillations with an effect on the all encompassing earth soul. This disrupted oscillation ratio could well be the trigger for the increasing disasters. It is not taken into consideration enough that it will not only hit the innocent but also the perpetrators when the world soul hits back.

Major damage is caused not only to the world soul when it comes to the dramatic forest fires such as in California, Greece or Spain. The aggrieved parties suffer emotional damage through these events, either directly or indirectly. One tries to extinguish the fires with great effort and often without quick success. Would it not be more sensible to create broad-based, large fire breaks where the fires cannot spread using corresponding instruments and in time?!

The whole magnitude of the destroyed world soul, respectively destroyed nature, manifests itself in the rising number of cancer cases and the related mortality. As body and soul are in correlation, the soul does not receive the necessary oscillations from the body to feel well. A long time ago one realised that unsolved psychic problems let the body fall ill, depending on the disrupted inter-oscillations and toxic state. Here, orthodox medicine speaks of psychosomatic illnesses. Approaching the dilemma with chemotherapeutics, instead of banking on nature, cannot be the goal. The creation of harmonious oscillations between body and soul should always stand in the foreground.

Foods have their own characteristic oscillations which have a harmonious effect on body and soul. Eating and drinking keep body and soul together. This piece of wisdom is well known. We are particularly partial towards some foods and others often have a dislike of it which no one can explain. If body and soul are imbalanced it is usually very sensible to eat a juice and raw vegetable diet. If this light food is eaten for up to 10 days, it has benefits for the heart. However, from the 11th day onwards, cardiac protein is broken down. The myocardial cells (myofibrils) are damaged! Physical wellbeing results in psychic harmony, which itself has an effect on the physical wellbeing. Such occasional fasting days therefore have a good effect on the correlation between body and soul. This results, not least, in psychic wellbeing and therefore the strength to deal much better with stress. If this strength is not there, no amount of psychic influence can help because the patient cannot implement a "conversational therapy" adequately in such an unfavourable state of mind. If the "psycho-patient" feels more comfortable all up, he will then be in a position to forgo psychotherapy more readily.

Psychotropic drugs are used too often and too fast and it is not taken into consideration enough that there is the danger of becoming addicted and the causes are not registered. This type of symptomatic therapy is often fraught with serious side effects.

No one should self-medicate with regard to physical-emotional health. In particular not with synthetic chemotherapeutics. It would be better to try it with plant preparations such as St. John's wort (hypericum perforatum), oats (avena sativa) and similar preparations. Herbal homeopathic remedies have no side-effects, however, and as opposed to chemotherapeutics, they have an advantageous radiation on the soul together with the good oscillations. It should, however, be noted that these herbal substances, e.g. St. John's wort, only start to act after three weeks.

The soul is also damaged during aircraft collisions. Relatives of the victims and the survivors of such disasters are marked for the rest of their life. Would it then not be more sensible if an international regulation came into force? Two aircraft, which are on a head-on approach, should not swerve up or down, but to the right! There would be no more aircraft collisions due to error, something which happened some years ago in Überlingen at Lake Constance. Much physical and emotional pain could be avoided for the persons concerned.

Another example of the psychic correlation with the body would be the shoulder-arm syndrome. One can repeatedly read the claim that shoulder-arm pain could only come from the emotional range. The people concerned "carry too much". A life situation is "too stressful" and "sits on the shoulders". Looked at in this way, every person with problems should also suffer from shoulder pain.

This is not the case. Primarily, toxins afflict the nerves which lead to the shoulders and arms. The nerves can no longer regulate blood flow so that less oxygen and nutrients reach the muscle cells and waste products are not transported off adequately. It also results in painful tension of the muscles. The tense muscles then subluxate (pull oblique), as a result so do the vertebral bodies, making the vertebral transverse processes press on the nerves. This closes the painful, vicious cycle. The soul is then affected by the oscillations originating from the pain syndrome. If we add events which burden the soul, more oscillation changes of the soul take place. The soul now acts on the material sector (shoulder-arm). And this closes the body-soul circle.

The necessary alternative is to polarise the nerves (for example with neural therapy), detox the organism and to loosen the muscle tensions. The disrupted oscillations will normalise and the soul will fell better again in the healthier body, provided no other reasons prevent healing. It must also be said that every person has certain tendencies towards weaknesses in the physical and emotional range.

The mysterious colours

Colours and their effect on the psyche play a role which should not be underestimated. Colours also have an effect on emotions, self-esteem and the immune system. Orange/Red, for example, have a stimulating effect. The colour deep blue conveys relaxing and calming feelings. Self-assurance is furthered by pine green. Yellow is said to have a pleasant and relaxing effect. Colours and physical wellbeing promote physical intensity and this again the faculty of belief.

An interesting point in this connection is the different gemstones with their oscillations, as well as the corresponding colours in connection with the star signs.

The Capricorn (22.12. to 20.1.) has the onyx and chrysopras as lucky stones. Its main colour is brown. If this colour shimmers towards red or gold, it gives the Capricorn a feeling of illustriousness.

Pisceans (20.2. to 20.3.) have the coral and amethyst as lucky stones. Their colour is grey. They try to loose the grey of inner loneliness all their life but are seldom successful in doing so.

Aquarians (21.1. to 19.2.) are assigned the gemstones amethyst, garnet and zirkonia. Their colour is indigo (blue colouring after violet), which they are very partial to.

Taureans (21.4. to 21.5.) react positively to the gemstone oscillations from turquoise, carneole and sapphire (natural stones). Green is their colour, which has a beneficial effect on the disposition and pleases them.

Aries (21.3. to 20.4.) has jaspis, heliotrope and diamond as lucky stones. The Aries' colour is red, it expresses courage and boldness.

Cancerians (22.6. to 22.7.) have the emerald, moon stone, scarab and pearl as their lucky gemstones: The colour white is pleasant for the calm and tranquil Cancerian and promotes wellbeing.

Geminis (22.5. to 21.6.) have chalcedon, chrysopras and agate as lucky stones. The colour yellow for the Gemini has a positive effect on the disposition, as well as being anti-spasmotic. They are also optimistic and harmonious in all manner of circumstances.

Virgos (24.8. to 23.9.) have the topaz, jaspis and carneole as their lucky stones. The colour blue reflects the balance and calm manner of the Virgo.

Leos (23.7. to 23.8) need the ruby and amber as their lucky stones. Orange is their colour. If the Leo has no time to dream, he will become slightly unpleasant and puts stress on his environment. He fears the unknown.

Scorpios (24.10. to 22.11.) have the agate, aquamarine and beryl as their lucky stones. The Scorpio loves the colour black as it underlines its mysterious manner and makes him interesting.

Libras (24.9. to 23.10.) require the aquamarine, opal, lapis lazuli and coral as lucky stones. The colour pink, the colour of harmony and beauty fits Libras best. It has a positive effect on its environment.

Sagittarians (23.11. to 21.12.) are enamoured by the royal colour purple. The turquoise is the lucky stone and the tiger eye is the auxiliary stone. Belief in the metaphysical and interest for the unusual characterise the Sagittarian and takes him from one extreme to the other. His optimism is always unbroken and he continuously tries to enthuse his fellow men.

The mysterious mind

Who doesn't know the saying "The spirit is willing but the flesh is weak"? Body-Soul-Mind is an entity born by oscillations. One finds few satisfying answers which sound logic to the question of what is the mind or spirit, how can one imagine it or what sort of entity is it. When, as the author believes, the soul is an energy formation of a specific type, the author also believes that the mind could be an energy formation, however of a somewhat different kind. The differentiation most surely lies in the frequencies of the energetic oscillations of the spirit. An unimaginably powerful energy with an unlimited intelligence in the whole cosmos, respectively universe, which we may be able to call God pulsates over the soul and spirit. An enormous energy, which has always been there from eternity to eternity. Without this enormous energy and its corresponding frequency there would most surely be no soul, no mind and no material phenomena, respective stars (suns) and planets. According to the laws of polarity, there must be a powerful negative energy as antithesis to the divine energy with its positive oscillations and frequencies. This negative energy, which is found throughout the whole universe, would therefore have to be looked at as the demonic. If a person is flooded with the civilisation toxins of our time, he tends more towards the negative direction with his thoughts. This is something which can only be improved when the excretory organs are strengthened and a reduction of the toxic concentration is possible. Removing toxins via the skin is an excellent support for the overall detox. The toxically-induced negativity is reinforced by the demonic cosmic energy in the concerned persons.

Our thoughts have energetic oscillations. Used correctly they can effect a lot in us and around us. Every person and every animal is surrounded by an aura which can be made visible with the so-called Kirlian method and which may represent the mind or spirit.

The existence of the spirit is comprehended more with our feelings than with the conscious mind. The spirit expresses itself in the famous attitude of mind, which is of utmost importance to manage all occurring problems. A good attitude comprises all positive feelings such as friendliness, happiness, practising love and patience, being tolerant towards the weaker, and in particular, consistently reminding oneself of charitableness. Good and constructive oscillations will be meted out to everyone whose mind is nourished by sympathy in the face of pain and suffering. Oscillations which emit from the mind reach the soul with which it is in correlation. The mind also acts on the material, where the brain stands in first place. It is assumed in general that the spirit is the thoughts, but it is oscillations produced in the material (brain) which in turn possess a metaphysical effect. This is confirmed adequately over and over again by the successes of the spiritual healers. Thoughts originate in the brain as a result of brain function. If a lot of people meet in a room (for example, a church) to jointly pray to God, it results in an enormous spiritual action with its oscillations and a positive overall effect. This overall effect is then beneficial in a reflexive manner for each individual. We have long kown that everything is oscillation and depends on the frequencies. Should we, one day, be successful in raising the atomic oscillations of our cells, we will be able to walk through walls.

An event comes to the author's mind where he still doesn't know whether it was a dream or reality. In March 1993, the author went to bed on time as usual. In the middle of the night, the author suddenly stood beside his bed with his face to the wall. The author was incredibly surprised because the toilet was located in the opposite direction. The night light spread a dim light so that when the author looked to the right, he saw his wife lying in bed. Then the author looked to the left, and saw a strong, thickset figure which, oddly enough, did not surprise him. The only thing the author also took note of was the grey, wrinkly skin. Today the author thinks that if it was not a dream, it could have been a space suit. At the next moment the author walked through the wall together with the being as if under an inner compulsion. The form and the action of going through the wall was so matter of fact as if the author had experienced it many times already. Having arrived in the courtyard, the author saw the neighbouring houses with their outside lights which let his garage appear in a bright light. Suddenly, a glaring white light overcame him and from then on, there is no memory of further perceptions.

A wise person once said that we only use approximately 10% of our mental capacity. Could it not be possible that we can raise the atomic oscillations of our cells with the residual 90% brain capacity so that we would be able to walk through walls or be capable of other deeds?

When referring to a world soul one should also take into consideration that there could be a world spirit just as well.

There could also be an overall spirit which forms from the oscillations of each individual in the case of a larger congregation of people who have met in an atmosphere of harmony. We are not yet able to attribute the spirit as phenomenon of scientific examinations with today's methods. According to experience, the scientific findings in many areas are continuously replaced with new ones which means that the old findings have been invalidated. That is why the total faith in science should be handled with great care.

It is more important to cultivate the empiricism of naturopathy which has developed over thousands of years. Approximately 170 people died during a landing approach in fog at Paris airport. The captain had activated the autopilot for the landing. The evaluation showed that it would have been safe to land the plane manually. According to media reports, however, the pilot had preferred to trust the approximately 36 on-board computers. The pilot's total belief in science cost the passengers their life. How far this just described case can be assigned to the mental law of series is anyone's guess.

A mysterious phenomenon strikes from time to time. On the one hand we experience a spade of plane crashes, then a continuance of train accidents, followed by a series of bus accidents, without being able to find a rational explanation for any of these. The attentive observer will also register this phenomenon in his or her environment to a small degree. Are these phenomena possibly caused by a world spirit and if yes, what irritates its oscillations and frequencies to cause such phenomena?

Perhaps physical influences also play a role. Mental learning steps, which result from the environment, most surely also influence the physical processes in accordance with the law of correlation between mind and body.

The overexploitation which has been taking place on earth for a long time and which leads to changes in the ecological balance, also changes the harmonious oscillations with their frequencies which the earth sends out and the world spirit absorbs accordingly. This reacts in a form less favourable for mankind, so that this creates an unfavourable correlation of the oscillations with their frequencies.

The mysterious subconsciousness

The subconsciousness acts on the mental level and expresses itself in feelings, sensations and also intuition, all of which are not tangible on a visible level. It seems as if each individual must acquire the understanding for the mental processes over and over again. One can look at the subconsciousness as an energy formation in a similar manner as one did with the soul and mind or spirit.

The spiritual healer programs his or her own subconsciousness and that of the patient via his/her power of belief. Disorders of the patient's body, which we call symptoms, are alleviated or removed by the subconsciousness which is involved in metabolic processes.

The law of realisation is mobilised with the power of thought. Independent of what we think, speak, do and feel, it represents an action. And this effects a reaction. If we influence our subconsciousness positively, the subconsciousness takes care of a positive reaction. However, if we think negatively, negative reactions will return to us.

What we perceive as true, be it negative or positive, the subconsciousness registers as a command which it obeys true to the intellectual laws. The mental imagination perceived as real, is decisive. That means, what I wish for, should pass off as fulfilled in my mental eye. The Bible quotes something very similar. Faith can move mountains, respectively if you believe you have received you will have already received.

The total subconsciousness of mankind is the result of the subconsciousness of each individual person. As the condition of all of mankind is more affected by toxins than we can imagine, thinking, as a rule, is also negative. In addition to the exposure to environmental toxins and the general electro-smog we have the toxic substances which are created in the body as a result of metabolism and which are even carcinogenic. It is therefore all the more important to strengthen the excretory organs with all available means and methods so that the body is detoxed well via these. Without strengthening the organism in its overall function, the chance of leading a happy existence is very low.

There have been too many people already who believed that one had to achieve everything through faith and who died after a certain period through organ failure or cancer. No doubt, symptoms (illnesses) will continue to be changed or removed through the power of faith. The causes which led to these, however, continued to exist and sooner or later new symptoms arose with a life of suffering or premature end. In a healthy body you can only have a healthy mind which feels well only then.

Too many people think negatively and so it is not surprising that the mass subconsciousness is overall negative. The goal should be to distance oneself from this and to call a positively reacting subconsciousness one's own. It is better to devote oneself to positive, happy thoughts in the morning, straight after waking up, than to harbour dark, negative thoughts. If someone sees everything from the blackest side early in the morning, the person will not feel well all day. Corresponding with the fact that most of the cell-regenerating hormones are formed during our before-midnight sleep, it is absolutely necessary to go to bed on time. If this is not possible because the heart causes problems, usually due to vegetative causes, one should practice natural sleep. To practise this, one should retire at about 6.30 p.m. read some relaxing literature and undertake the relaxing trip through the body, then sleep until one awakes. One should then rise immediately and do some activity. As soon as one feels tired again, return to sleep until 6.30 or 7 a.m. This creates a good alternating oscillation between body and subconsciousness so that the person will fell better altogether. After lunch, it is advisable to take a rest between 2 and 2.30 p.m. in accordance with the biorhythm. However, one should not sleep during this time, so that welcome tiredness can arrive at around 7 p.m. It is possible that success will not show immediately, but a corresponding perseverance will surely be rewarded.

Hypnotic treatment brought the existence of the subconsciousness to light a long time ago. Events which were not known, showed up to be stored in the subconsciousness. These processes were then activated by hypnosis. It therefore also stands to reason that events from earlier lives are also stored in the subconsciousness.

A young woman had a traffic accident where her car was a total write-off. This weighed so heavily on her subconsciousness that her resistance dropped and the pre-cancerosis tests according to Prof. Neunhoeffer, Dr. Scheller and Dr. Gutschmidt rose. After the shock and damage had been dealt with, the pre-cancerosis values fell again and there was only little activity to be seen in the laboratory analyses. This case clearly shows that defence processes in the body are co-influenced by the subconsciousness.

A Japanese scientist has found that water also reacts to positive and negative oscillations. A drop of water looked at under the microscope changed its molecular structure to the most beautiful shapes when positive, divine truths were thought during the examination. By contrast, the drop of water changed to a distorted image when the observer influenced his subconsciousness through negative thoughts during the microscopic examination.

The subconsciousness represents a mighty switching station in the life of a person. In his writings, a great philosopher[3] pointed out that every person will need an alternative practitioner or doctor at some stage. It has often happened, that a cancer patient refrained from all treatment and visited a therapist who wanted to conquer the cancer with stones and their radiation. To use only this measure alone harbours the great risk of not receiving adequate therapy. While conducting the stone radiation therapy there is great danger that important time passes by unused if immunotherapeutic measures are disregarded. It may work now and then but the risk is incomparably higher. Moreover, the issue is not programming the subconsciousness, but first and foremost the intensity of the emotion-dependent ability to believe. But even if it exists, today's prevailing environmental pollution and its related multi-intoxication must not be ignored. Healthy body, healthy soul and a healthy consciousness effect a successful subconsciousness. According to cosmic laws, we attract good events when the thoughts are activated in a positive direction and are charged with feeling. In the opposite case, unpleasant events will come into our life, when we send out negative thoughts with the desctructive effects. The subconsciousness transforms all mental activities into the respective events. We should let our thoughts run free before going to sleep and imagine our wishes as having already been fulfilled by the subconsciousness[4]. It is crucial here to charge our wishful thoughts with feeling and intense belief. However, before any action, it is also of great importance to be clear about what we actually want. We should remember that more power lies in good thoughts than in negative perceptions. Congeneric good souls seek each other and are brought together on earth.

An old truism says that the same perceptions effect the same results. It is advantageous to greet the day happily in the morning and to imagine an energetic protective corona around the people close to us, similar to a halo. We also subconsciously program our subconsciousness with our perceptions. It is recommended to only wish every person the very best. It returns to us sooner or later and shows us repeatedly that the good is stronger than the evil.

A great malady in many marriages is the pathological criticism of the partner. The criticising partner doesn't do him/herself or the partner any good, when the criticism isn't really justified. No person stands above the other because at the beginning and end of life we are all the same. According to the law of the cosmos, burdening the subconsciousness of the other in such a manner will act on the originator. When a partnerhip ends, there will always be good memories of the part of the joint path which two partners have trodden and this should be upheld with gratitude. The subconsciousness with its oscillations and frequencies should reflect this in a positive manner. The alternating oscillations between the conscious and subconsciousness can be compared to the vegetative system. If one part outweighs, the vegetative system is unbalanced which then leads to disruptions in the supply of the organ systems. The sympathetic trunk, for example, excites and narrows the vessels. The opponent is the parasympathetic trunk with its inhibiting and vessel-distending effect. The vagus is the third component which, as the tenth cranial nerve, extends all the way to the solar plexus and, to a greater extent, also possesses parasympathetic effects. Here too, we have the correlation of the overall vegetative system with the subconsciousness. The subconsciousness reacts similar to a computer chip, which displays what has been entered on it. The subconsciousness cannot decide whether this is good or bad. It only ever mirrors what it has been given. If someone tries to analyse the good and bad, that person will easily slide into a troublesome uncertainty. According to the law of polarity, both are part of life. Trying to remove the bad would turn out to be an ineffectual attempt right from the beginning. If one part were missing, the other part could not be identified. We know of the operating mode of the good and subconsciously enjoy this, as the bad is unpleasant for us due to its aura, or vibes. Mankind is automatically drawn towards the good, similar to light and shade, where we are not able to remove the shade. The light displaces shade or also darkness. That is why we should not despair when the blows of fate trouble us. If we nurture the hope for change to a pleasing development, we will, after passing through the bottom of a valley, come to an elevation point earlier or later which bears the change towards the good in it. The change from high to low promotes our inner further development. The more the subconsciousness is influenced in the positive direction, the more it looks after bringing a happy turn to life. The fact that there is good and bad does not mean that we have to accept the bad (or evil). Mankind can decide freely to accept the bad or the good.

There are many people who - subconsciously - already came to know the effect of the subconsious in their childhood. How often have we had the situation before an examination that it could not be managed. And then it actually turned out badly. In contrast, it usually turned out well even under the most difficult conditions when the subconsciousness had been programmed with the conviction of success. Sometimes success comes quicker and at other times it takes longer. It depends on how intensely and emotionally and with how strong an ability to believe the subconsciousness is programmed.

As a child, the author often thought of Tahiti and dreamt of the Wild West. He wanted to become a Western rider and cowboy and ride in the prairie. The mother, to whom he repeatedly raved about the Wild West as a thirteen-year old, warned him of the dangers. Many years were still to pass before he landed on Bora Bora/Tahiti in May of 1985. In 2001 he then travelled with one of his daughters to the Wild West to Tombstone/ Arizona. There they underwent training as cowboy and Western rider with examination and certificate. The author only heard about the mental laws of attraction in action in 1976 within the scope of the naturopathy studies, when writings from Dr. Murphy were recommended. As a child, the author had known nothing of the laws of action and reaction and subconsciously imagined his dreams as fulfilled. The author then didn't further activate his perceptions for many years, otherwise the realisation of his dreams would not have taken so long. The case was similar with the Tahiti trip which also resulted some decades later. The author's father was a miner in those days, the place of employment being far away from the family. The author was always happy when he could visit his father during the school holidays. When he undertook a stroll through the city close-by, he saw a small accordion in a music shop.

The author was about eleven years old and thought that he could play the instrument without much ado. He asked his father to buy the accordion for him. The author answered the father's question, whether he could actually play it, in the affirmative because he was convinced that he would be able to do so. They then entered the music shop and bought the accordion. Back at home, the author was to play something. The author quickly picked up the accordion and wanted to press the keys and buttons. But before he cold produce the first sound, he received a slap in the face. The reason being that he had worn the instrument the wrong way round. The keys were on the left side and the basses on the right side. The father then took up the accordion and played the song "Schön ist so ein Ringelspiel" (That's the beauty of a merry-go-round). Until then, the author had not known that he could play. The author's daughter had a similar experience in the Wild West, when he played Western songs on a mouth organ around the camp fire. She also had no inkling of this. In the following period he began to practice the song "Komm mit mir nach Tahiti" (Come to Tahiti with me) with one finger on the instrument. It was the first try on this instrument and every time he later played this song, he imagined the South Sea Island with the bizarre mountains and the blue ocean all around. The author repeatedly programmed his subconsciousness in this way without knowing about the effectiveness of the same which had then taken care of the realisation some decades later. People differ from other people by their expressions, be this by gestures, facial expression or in their behaviour. This happens subconsciously, respectively without involvement of the conscious. Many a person takes on an image which is taken on and reinforced by the subconsciousness. This is how oscillations are created with the respective frequencies, which are subconsciously registered by the opposite party. If these oscillations are good, it creates affection. If the oscillations are unfavourable, the other party perceives the radiation as unpleasant and the person is classified as unpleasant. Sometimes a person's body language expresses security or insecurity which is often reflected by a crossing of the arms by the other person during a discussion.

The subconscious behaviours of people are as different as their faces. Each individual will be perceived by his neighbour depending on type and disposition. Some people appear to be self-assured without being so, others appear insecure without being so in his innermost. Very often a certain behaviour is provoked, which would otherwise not be expressed. If someone finds his life okay, he has achieved a lot in his psychological development. If a person asks himself where he comes from, who he really is and where the trip to eternity will take him, he is looking for the reference to his personality because he may be frightened of loosing his identity. The hope of being able to reach a better life drives many contemporaries to undreamt-of activities. On the search for insights, the searching person goes through feelings of apprehensions, existing prejudices and is in danger, via aggression, of lastly falling into apathy or indifference. Another person would like to be more than he is and uses a whole plethora of status symbols for this purpose. If this doesn't arouse the attention of others, the person will loose himself in a great dissatisfaction with his life. The emotions so important for the subconsciousness fall by the wayside so that nothing much can really change towards the positive in his life.

The mysterious consciousness

We are aware of innumerous things. Our environment communicates itself to us in many variations which we comprehend with our 5 senses. The healthier a person is, the more he will experience life consciously. This again depends very much on his brain function and this on the whole organism whose organs, in their correlation, are supposed to enable a well-functioning metabolism.

So many things come into our consciousness from the past, the present and the future. The less a person's health is afflicted and the person feels well, the more he is able to live consciously. A person who is constantly exposed to a flurry of activity, stress and other burdens and who therefore cannot collect his wits, lives outside of his life. Most people only become aware of this when they have missed everything, when they experience the rest of their life old and sick. Blaming others for their misery or complaining all the time doesn't help either. Perhaps one or the other, when looking back on his life consciously, will recognise the errors to be found in the way he lived his life. As it is never too late to change, many could still turn the boat around and consciously create a positive lifestyle of awareness. The materially thinking person usually only focuses on the material and has lost the relationship with nature.

Of course one cannot live without the necessary small change which is necessary to upkeep one's needs in life. However, everyone should be aware that money is only a symbol and, like everything else, is subject to a cycle. To hang on to it consciously and hoard it means blocking the money flow, respectively the cycle. Our water, ground products and the good quality of our air have already been sacrificed to the general greed, as has the health and life of many people.

The flooding of all areas of life with toxins makes it ever harder to live an easy-going and conscious life. A moderate lifestyle promotes the perception of harmony and brings on feelings of happiness. Instead of consciously developing a good inner life, mankind is constantly getting further away from inner values with this superficial lifestyle.

Despite the development of total technology and electronics, which makes it easier and quicker to deal with many things, people have less and less time. The day is over quickly, as is the week, the month, the year.

Most people lack a consciousness of time. To restore this lost consciousness of time, everyone should recall the day in his mind's eye before falling asleep. The time is always the same but how we use it and consciously feel it, depends on our inner attitude.

Everyone is able to bring existing conditions into consciousness with the power of his thoughts. It is necessary to learn to let go if one wants to develop a good consciousness. It is also necessary to free oneself of competitive behaviour and negative thoughts. First, it is necessary to try and change oneself in a positive direction. We cannot change our fellow men, only proceed with good example by reviewing our behaviour and integrating it into our consciousness. A person thinks too much of all sorts of things, for example what has to be done next. It would be more important to live the moment consciously. Developing conscious gratitude for the momentary situation and being pleased with it. In particular, when there is no pain or disabled mobility, the person feels well all up and is grateful for this. During the work which is currently being undertaken one should not start thinking about all pending problems. Concentrating on the work at hand definitely takes priority. Success grows from the concentration on what has to be done for the respective task. The sense of achievement arises from the conscious activity with the resultant success. This creates the happiness and therefore the positive oscillation on mind and soul. No matter what someone does, the issue is to feel consciously. If someone takes a break during work, it is more important to relax than to make plans and be at the next task with one's thoughts. Creative ideas can originate particularly in a relaxed state. If situations occur which require full application of body and mind, spontaneous solutions often develop which appeared impossible earlier on. Of course this depends on how constructive and capable of development the thoughts are. Destructive thoughts attract failures and prevent realistic spontaneous solutions. To be able to make the right decisions, the thoughts must be projected towards the realistic processes. Proceedings must correspond with the truth to be able to decide correctly. Physically and mentally weak people like to avoid problem solving as they prefer to shirk responsibility. However, it is the unsolved problems which are particularly burdening. A person who is physically healthier finds it easier to face problems consciously. It is therefore important to detox the body over and over again and strengthen the excretory organs. Being physically fit also means occasionally showing your "teeth" when unjustified attacks occur. This helps the growth of confidence in us and our existing skills. Who would not like to go through life without having constant apprehensions. The healthier a person is, the sooner he is able to develop feelings of happiness.

We often do the wrong thing and are annoyed afterwards when negative events occur in our life. That is why decisions should be made consciously and well thought out. This is not always easy. Our pets are better off in this regard as they follow their instincts. We however, must approach all problems consciously if we wish to solve them to our own satisfaction. To do this, it is necessary to stay open-minded in all directions. Without confidence in our own skills and talents, we move in a circle from which it is very difficult to escape. If we succeed in becoming conscious of the driving truths of peace, harmony and love, an important step in the right direction has been undertaken. Developing the consciousness for biological nutrition over and over again is an overall help in perceiving life in a pleasant manner.

Consciousness as summation of brain function with its neuro-metabolism gives us the opportunity of consciously grasping and experiencing our whole.

Riding is a splendid experience for a horse lover. While the Western rider practices violence-free riding, the English rider practices deadening his feelings towards his horse. To make the horse obey tournament riders, in particular, use a bridle, a painful experience for the horse. Quite a few riders use a razor-sharp snaffle for this purpose. The horse does not have a pain sound and obeys the rider under pain. The Western rider guides his horse in a painless manner by shifting weight without tearing around in the horse's mouth. If he doesn't ride without a bridle he gives the change of direction some emphasis by a slight pull on the reins, without hurting the horse. Every horse lover should become aware of this. People who are in involved in "bullfighting" lack the awareness that it is not really a fight, but an animal torturing slaughter. While the riders on horseback attack the bull with their lances, the torero pushes one sword after the other into the bull's back until it breaks down covered in blood and in inhuman pain. A prohibition of the so-called "bullfight" would be welcome. There are many examples of cruelty to animals where the respective government should make an end of it. A change of consciousness in favour of the animals is necessary. We can change given conditions with consciousness, provided the relevant people use their consciousness accordingly.

It is necessary to turn our thoughts into the right direction. Conscious thinking deposits in the unconscious and automatically effects a correlation. Infectious diseases afflict animals because they are not kept species-appropriate and this weakens their defence system. Then one pumps cortisone and antibiotics into the animals so they can be sold quickly, without thinking that people will also become sicker as a result of the consumption cycle. A healthy consciousness for the wellbeing of man and animal should develop here very soon.

Some time ago, the author visited a thermal bath. While swimming in the soothing warm water, he sensed a strange, light tingling on the skin. Of course he immediately started to think about the reason for this and had the idea of checking the pH value of the water. He found an indicator paper in his swimming bag which is used to check the urine pH. He was very surprised that the paper strip, which he held into the thermal water, turned yellow instead of colouring into the blue range. According to the Uralyt-U test strip, the blue range indicates the alkaline pH of 6.8 to 8.0 while the yellow colour of the test strip indicated a pH of approx. 5.6. As the thermal bath also had an indoor pool, the author repeated the procedure in the pool and the test strip also turned yellow. He became aware that he may be swimming around in an acidic environment. This disturbed him extremely. He then went under the shower and held the test strip into the running water. The test strip from the Uralyt-U package turned blue, respectively into the alkaline range. If it turns out that thermal water has a pH of 5.0-5.5 it is recommended to follow this with an alkaline bath in the tub. As far as is known, thermal water is supposed to be full of minerals. Minerals have a de-acidifying and alkaline effect. How is it then possible that the pH value was around 5.5 in the thermal bath the author visited. Could it be the chlorine or another substance which over-acidified the water? As we absorb through the skin, we take acid in this case.

The mysterious body

Our body contains not only organs, nerves and muscles but also our soul and mind or spirit. If disorders occur in the body, the soul and mind also suffer. A sick body does not produce harmonious oscillations. It has been demonstrated over and over again that even serious fateful events in a person's life can be coped with easier when the concerned person is healthy and resistant. As we know, everything is oscillation. Even matter oscillates at a frequency that we cannot perceive. The body, soul and mind are in a certain oscillating relationship, depending on how healthy or sick a person is. Treating the body with so-called "cures" which stress it and, while directed against a symptom, cause new disorders cannot be the answer to everything. Environmental pollution, electro-smog and genetically manipulated food all on their own are already enough. One hears little of the geopathic zones (interference zones on the earth's surface) which are an additional stress factor for us, and where many a sleeping place is to be found. It is particularly tragic when an unfavourable earth radiation has an intensified effect on the human body through water veins and damages it. Some animals, in particular dogs, have the ability to avoid radiation polluted sites. Cats, by contrast, look for places which are radiation exposed and feel comfortable there. When the wife of a sprightly pensioner died of cancer, he had their bed checked with a divining rod. Above the wife's bed the divining rod showed geopathic stress from head to toe. On the husband's side, stress was only detected in the head section. Six months after the measurement, the pensioner showed Alzheimer symptoms. The man became incapable of acting in law within a very short period and has been a care case since because his memory failed completely. The so-called global grid knots (cancer zones) every 2.5 m are deemed as particularly dangerous. Building biologists or radiesthesia experts determine where radiation-free sites are located in the house so that the beds can be placed there, if possible. A fine particle measurement should be conducted at this opportunity, as well as a test for fungal spores in the house.

If an acidosis (over-acidification) is added to geopathic stress, the situation is not very favourable for the person concerned.

However, it is not possible to do without any acids at all in the organism as it needs these to gain energy. Every cell produces energy as a result of metabolism. The cell also needs neutral fats (triglycerides), which are introduced into the cells, to produce energy. The body also needs L-carnitine, which is formed from methionine and lysine. Magnesium also has to be available so that adenosine triphosphate can be changed to adenosine diphosphate. The split-off phosphate part is an energy molecule which is deemed as essential in the body's whole energy requirement. If there is too much acid in the body, the haemoglobin (blood pigment) cannot bind enough oxygen so that the cells do not receive enough oxygen. Chlorine, phosphorus and sulphur have a negative electrical charge and are therefore classed as minerals which form acid. The bases are the antithesis with a calming and harmonising effect. Hormones and enzymes regulate all processes in the organism. However, a slightly base environment is needed so that the enzymes can fulfil their functions. Iron, potassium, sodium and calcium, for example, have a positive electrical charge and are therefore classed as base-forming cell function substances. Today, it is most likely the privilege of indigenous peoples to maintain the biological balance. That is why they are not familiar with the diseases of civilisation with all their disastrous effects. They are also not aware that strong over-acidification gelatinises the blood and tissue fluid and makes it viscous. The red blood cells become immobile, thus reducing capillary blood flow. Many a heart attack or stroke was due to strong over-acidification.

Minerals are dissolved from bones and teeth to allow de-acidification, if this suffices by that stage.

Many a disc damage is also due to over-acidification.

Hair loss is often a result of over-acidification as the hair follicles are not adequately covered by the micro-circulation. The red blood corpuscles are immobile and do not penetrate the smallest hair vessels. There is a lack of oxygen and nutrients, often accompanied by a zinc deficiency or a strong overload of the body with toxins.

Sciatica is triggered when, for example, acidic waste is stored on the nerves. Tendons, ligaments and tissue loose their elasticity and are therefore also subject to a strong loss of elasticity. The body fluids circulate sluggishly when white sugar, which makes the blood sluggish, is consumed in addition. With its high concentration it cannot be absorbed adequately by the cells, especially when permeability of the cell membranes often no longer functions. Brown cane sugar with its lower percentage concentration is suitable for entering the cells where it is also processed. Diseases and early ageing are the result of the overall toxic stress which generally receives too little attention. With increasing frequency one hears of small children having strokes. One can hardly talk about age-related deposits in the vessels. If the excretory organs work with a reduced output, the "garbage bin" (body) becomes fuller and fuller so that some people can no longer think clearly due to the intoxication.

It is particularly important for every person to drink a teaspoonful of base powder dissolved in half a litre of water around 3 p.m. and to eat as many vegetables and uncooked vegetarian food as possible. This measure often effects a surprising improvement of the mental state. It is certain that stressed people are in a permanent negative mood, which has lots of side effects. The question arises why so many (psycho)therapists don't also take care of the organs and toxic pollution of their patients and therefore have so many therapeutic failures! It should certainly have done the rounds by now that nearly all illnesses, respectively civilisation disorders, are triggered by intoxication (toxic stress). The oscillations on mind and soul are corresponding and are reflected back from there to the body.

How toxically polluted do people have to be who attack and murder fellow students without cause. Usually they contribute increasingly to a misjudgement of their situation through their lifestyle.

Many a frenzied killer often suffers from a not always perceptible precancerosis (pre-cancerous stage), something which seriously increases the general intoxication. There are early cancer detection tests to determine this (according to Prof. Neunhoeffer, Dr. Scheller and Dr. Gutschmidt), which have been developed by a physician, a pharmacist and a professor and which hardly attract attention in medicine. These tests are ignored by orthodox medicine because the health insurances do not take care of the costs. Orthodox medicine as emergency and substitute medicine or in the case of vital operations is, unfortunately, unable to strengthen the patients' organs and defence system. This is only possible by means of holistic therapy as explained, for example in the book "Healthy or exhausted? Holistic therapy/Naturopathy" by Wolfgang Rietig (BOD Verlag Norderstedt, Germany). It is time that the prescriptions from non-medical practitioners and naturopaths are approved and paid for. Public health would, most assuredly, be better and there would be fewer extreme offenders in future, who attack teachers and students with their minds totally diseased. One needs to remember that many people have financial restrictions and often cannot afford natural remedies and treatments. Biologic food and local, untreated fruit should be subsidised so that not as much sprayed and irradiated food would have to be bought.

As a result of the toxic load, the impulses at the synapse (connection of the nerve cells) do not jump adequately from one cell to the other as the formation of transmitting substances is hindered by the toxic load. This inevitably leads to fear, depression and/or aggressive behaviour. The performance of the afflicted person usually drops and he becomes very sensitive towards his environment, withdraws or reacts with downright violence. Due to the permanent negative mood he is in, the person naturally has unfavourable vibes for his fellow men. They avoid this person. Friends, acquaintances and sometimes also relatives increasingly turn away from this person. The hatred of the frenzied attacker, for example, builds up until it discharges and innocent fellow students, teachers and other people are attacked, threatened or murdered. The state totally abandons the concerned persons in this situation.

The cell and future of each country, the family, is not paid enough attention. However, it would be especially necessary here to invest a higher financial backing. Parents must have more time for their children again. Children need attention, care, recognition and security and should not be placed in day care centres where there is no parental attention. This is the only way unfavourable developments can be counteracted. The self-confidence of a child grows and its development is turned into orderly paths. One parent should have the opportunity of taking care of the children at home without having to endure economic disadvantages! This takes a load off the parental educator and the parent is far more resilient against stress and can respond better to its child.

In addition, it is more necessary than ever before to increase school psychologists and also to employ more teachers. The teacher is better able to deal with the individual student and his or her personal circumstances when the classes are smaller.

The author is of the opinion, that teachers should be delegated to shooting associations (gun clubs), so that they can protect themselves and the students against the frenzied attackers, as he will usually only end his attacks when he runs out of ammunition or is hindered from committing further attacks by police action. There would then definitely be fewer or no fatalities. Instead of closing more and more police stations one should open new ones, increase salaries and staff them with more personnel. This would also be a benefit to the general safety of the citizens.

The police are, in general, understaffed, poorly paid and not always able to be at a scene immediately when this is required. And so one leaves the children, who are the future of the nation, to their fate. The rooms in the schools should be closed during lessons and security personnel should patrol the hallways. Entry to the school should be regulated by security gates and detector controls.

The safety of children should not depend on money. The German Federal Court of Audit has repeatedly acknowledged that around 30 billion Euros are wasted annually. The government should reduce this squander to zero and use it to ensure the security of children and teachers.

In the sense of a continuously rising intoxication in the environment it is important to know that, in the course of our lives, we channel about 40-50 kg toxins through our body. The result of this is that the annual cancer mortality rises constantly. Chronic diseases are also on the increase. However, before each therapy comes the diagnosis and this starts with the anamnesis.

Which operations has the patient undergone or which diseases of civilisation has he experienced?

How were the progress and the recovery time of these processes? Which constitution does the patient have?

Is he tall or short? What does the patient weigh, is he slim or overweight and/or bloated? There are billions of people on this world and yet each one is different. The same applies to illnesses and their progress. In this context the question, which illnesses or complaints the patient is currently exposed to is also important.

How is the blood pressure at which time of day?

It is best to measure blood pressure on the upper arm but it only provides information about the current pressure ratios in the body's blood vessels. One should remember that the blood pressure can be within the normal range but the heart can be just short of a fail-ure. Whether blood pressure is high or low depends mainly on the cardiac function, where however, hormone release in the adrenal glands and the sympathetic trunk (stimulating part of the vegetative system) play a role which should not be underestimated.

If the function of the adrenal glands is irritated through inflammation or other illnesses, there can be an increase or decrease in the release of hormones which is then reflected in high or low blood pressure. A good ECG doesn't necessarily mean good cardiac performance as is generally and erroneously assumed. The ECG only records the energetic lead and not the force of myocardial contraction. No long-term ECG can go past this fact either!

Orthodox medicine is in a dilemma here, which should change sooner or later when the new blood test N – terminal pro BNT to determine the force of myocardial contraction has been declared fail-safe.

Dysrhythmias are a typical effect of intoxication, although the heart may be strong. In this case there is stress on the sinus node (pace maker) in the right atrium. If the sinus node with its approximately 72 beats/min. fails, the Aschoff-Tawara node with a rhythm of approx. 45 actions per minute takes over. Should the Aschoff-Tawara node then fail as a result of excessive damage due to toxins, the bundle of His, with approximately 12 beats per minute, takes over supply of the heart with the rhythm impulses, which effect the cardiac actions. In the past, many a person was buried alive when the physician or the examiner did not register the 12 beats per minute. Many apparent dead had hairs in the bones of their hands which they had torn out before they suffocated after regaining consciousness. Before their death many people ordered that they wanted a Baunscheidt's treat-ment. If the pustules erupted on the skin, the apparently dead person was still alive and escaped this fate.

If, however, there is an attack-like weakness of the cardiac vessels, a heart attack is the usual course of things. In this case, the offer of blood for the heart is not adjusted to the requirement. Unclear pain in the left chest, left arm, especially along the inner side all the way to the small finger indicates a looming heart attack. The left abdominal region is sometimes involved as is the left shoulder. These are often accompanied by inner unrest fear and attacks of sweating. These alarm signals should be checked out immediately in an emergency hospital.

The following is also to be said with regard to the cardiac insufficiency. While measuring the blood pressure, one should record the heart rate at the 5th intercostal space with the stethoscope and stop watch. Then one should count the pulse waves for one minute with the stop watch. Each ejection of blood from the heart arrives as a pulse wave at the wrist. Therefore, the same number of pulse waves and heart beats has to be recorded. If fewer pulse waves arrive at the wrist than heart beats are counted, it means that the heart beats but it does not eject blood. And this means cardiac insufficiency as it beats empty, by not ejecting any blood. Every therapist worth his salt will do this examination at each consultation or in the case of cardiac complaints. If the left cardiac muscle is weak, blood will back up in the lung. This means that a person cannot breathe through fully when on an ascent or walking quickly up to the 3rd floor of a house. This sometimes leads to a collection of fluid in the lung. As everything in the body is controlled by way of hormones and enzymes, a thyroid function test in the laboratory should not be neglected. In the practice, one should record the basal metabolic rate by way of blood pressure amplitude and pulse rate per minute via Read's formula as a quick determination of the over/under or normal function.

The heart sends out centrifugal oscillations which can cause pain in peripheral tissue. In earlier times one believed that the heart was the seat of the soul. Many people gain weight although they eat little. They usually suffer an insufficiency of the right cardiac muscle. The blood collects in the venous system and from there in the lymph system. Blood and lymph fluid enter into the tissue as the vessels extend. Homeopathic remedies, which act on the right cardiac muscle as well as on the elastic fibres and connective tissue, are indicated here.

Cardiac activity is subject not only to intoxication but also the vegetative nervous system. On the one hand we have the stimulating part (sympathetic trunk) and on the other the inhibiting part, the parasympathetic trunk. These two parts should be in balance. In addition we have the vagus nerve, which extends from the brain all the way to the pit of the stomach and has its function in that region.

A well functioning organism needs blood vessels which should be free of plaque and damage. One of the strongest causes of arteriosclerosis is not only raised blood fat values but also rheumatism as expression of a masked tuberculosis and syphilis. These factors cause inflammatory processes on the blood vessels. In the case of diabetes patients, the arteriosclerosis mainly hits the coronary vessels as well as the cerebral vessels. There is also danger of arteriosclerosis if high blood pressure persists over a longer period, something which is generally known.   Nicotine damages the coronary arteries and the arteries of the legs in the same manner. A diet high in fats and proteins is a major contributor towards arteriosclerosis. Vegetarian whole foods are the alternative here.

Mental stress and emotional or psychological conflicts lead to an unfavourable correlation between body, mind and soul. Supporting the body with its functions is the motto, as is positive thinking. Thorough examinations in various directions are necessary for this. The good expert will not only tap the spine, do a hip joint test and tap the renal beds, indeed he will also look for facial signs. Measuring the blood pressure and determining the heart rate are obligatory. A urine test in the practice and laboratory blood tests round off the overall picture. Early cancer detection according to Prof. Dr. Neunhoeffer, the carcinochrome test according to Dr. Gutschmidt and also the Dr. Scheller test (blood smear under the microscope) are necessary examinations. Many an unexplained illness has its causes in an early stage of cancer and the result is high intoxication of the body. This then results in organ damage. The bioelectronic function diagnostic according to Dr. Voll[5] is necessary to arrive at a good diagnosis. After all, there could be weaknesses or inflammatory processes which necessitate a specific therapy. According to Dr. Voll it is necessary to measure the AP points not only next to the nails but also 3-4 parts on the organ meridian. Sole measurement next to the foot or hand nails is of no value as only one organ part will be covered by this. For example, the circulation meridian next to the nail only covers the arteries. The veins follow as second measuring point and the third acupuncture point is for the coronary arteries. The measuring points of the organ parts can be seen in the Hand-Foot diagram.

Foot

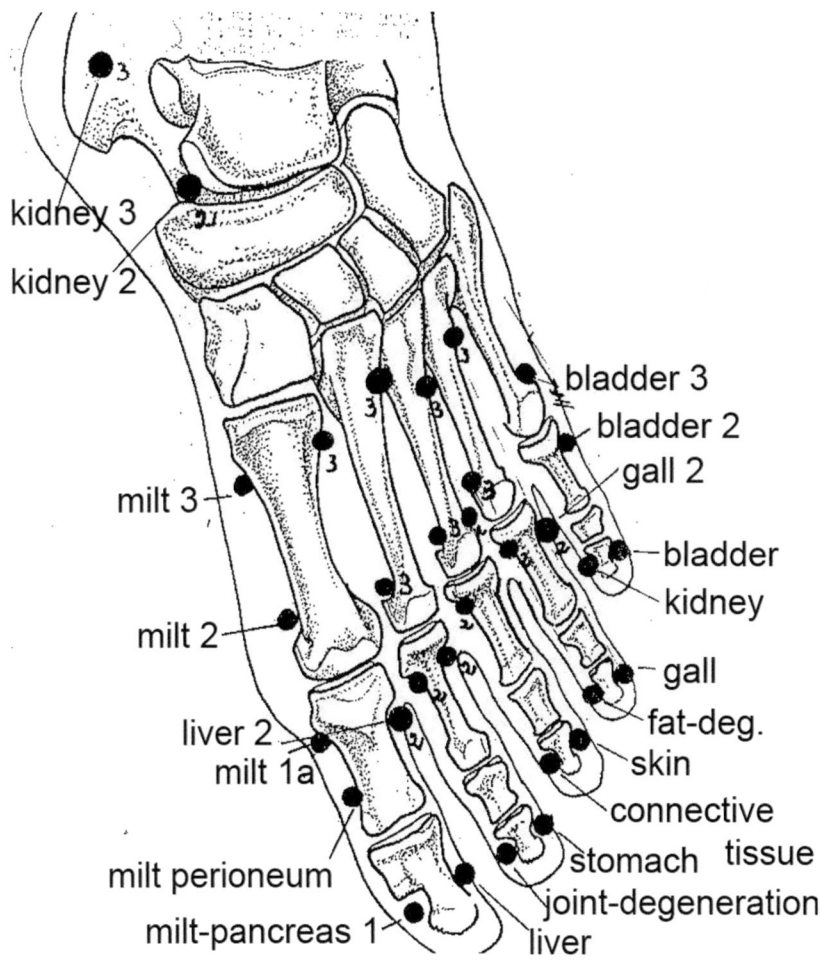

kidney 3

kidney 2

milt 3

milt 2

liver 2

milt 1a

milt perioneum

milt-pancreas 1

bladder 3

bladder 2

gall 2

bladder

kidney

gall

fat-deg.

skin

connective tissue

stomach

joint-degeneration

liver

Hand

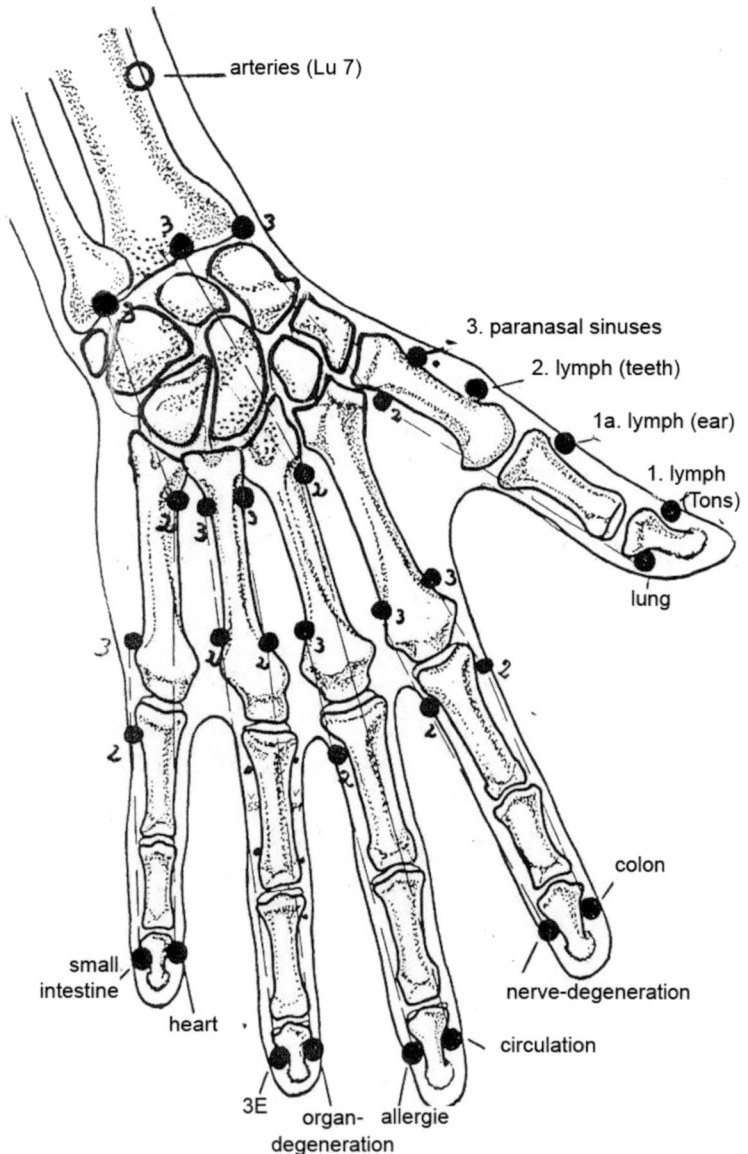

arteries (Lu 7)

3. paranasal sinuses

2. lymph (teeth)

1a. lymph (ear)

1. lymph (Tons)

lung

colon

nerve-degeneration

circulation

small intestine

heart

3E

organ-degeneration

allergie

Energy perfusion

Energy perfusion with a BFD unit according to Dr. Voll also represents an electro-physical treatment. In the case of total perfusion, two foot electrodes are connected with each other, as well as two hand styluses and these are connected to the unit via the plus socket. The forehead electrode left and right are connected by a cable which is connected to the minus socket. One can conduct a total perfusion with a quenching frequency of 0.4 and 12 Hz. This is then followed by some fixed frequencies which influence various illnesses:

Indication	Frequency in Hz	Active electrode on red connector (+)	Passive electrode on black connector (-)
Angina	9.45	Plate electrode on the side of neck with stronger complaints	Plate electrode on the opposite side of the neck
Angina pectoris	9.45	Moisten plate electrode if necessary with magnesium chloride solution and place on heart region	Plate electrode on the back
Fear	5.8	One hand electrode into the left hand	One hand electrode into the right hand
Arteriosclerosis	3.3	For blood pressure with long, hard arterial murmur which is heard in the bend of the elbow when measuring blood pressure. When this noise disappears and the blood pressure drops it is a sign that the spasm has gone as a result of treatment and that treatment can be concluded	
Arthritis	9.6	Attach a plate electrode to the front or outer side of the joint	Attach the counter electrode to the rear or inner side of the joint
Bladder complaints	9.4	Foot electrode underneath the foot of the side with the stronger complaints	Foot electrode under the other foot

Bron-chitis	9.4	Hand electrode	Foot electrode
Dysme-nor-rhoea	3.5 +1.9	Hand electrode	Hand electrode
Dysme-nor-rhoeic bleeding	4.0	Hand electrode	Hand electrode
Endo-crine Disorder	9.45 9.5	Hand electrode	Hand electrode Dysfunctions of the adrenal gland Dysfunctions of the thyroid gland Dysfunctions of the gonad Dysfunctions of the pituitary gland
Joint mobilisa-tion	9.6	Compare arthritis	
Joint pain from gout	9.4	Attach electrodes as for circulatory problems	
Hoarse-ness	9.5	Plate electrode on the larynx	Plate electrode in the neck
High blood pressure	6.0 9.2 9.4	Hand electrode Systolic high pressure: hyperto-nia and extra systoles Diastolic high pressure: kidney damage, diabetes and chronic eczema Spastic high pressure	Hand electrode
Hyper-tonia arterios-clerotic	3.3	Hand electrode	Hand electrode

Hyper-tonia diastolic	9.2	Hand electrode	Hand electrode
Hyper-tonia climacteric	9.5	Hand electrode	Hand electrode
Hypertonia spastic	9.45	Hand electrode	Hand electrode
Sciatica	9.7	a) one sided sciatica: 1. active foot electrode when the neuritic complaints are on the lower thigh and foot, passive plate electrode on back of upper thigh. 2. active plate electrode over spine in the lumbar region when lumbar sections of the sciatic nerve are involved. Foot electrode as passive electrodes. b) both sided sciatica active foot electrodes, inactive plate electrodes onto lumbar region: three-electrode treatment for longitudinal supply of both extremities.	
Inflammation of periosteum	2.65	Plate electrode on the inflamed part	Hand or foot electrode, depending on location of periostitis
Laryngitis	9.5	Plate electrode on the larynx	Plate electrode on the neck
Menstruation, heavier bleeding	2.5	Vaginal electrode	Foot electrode or hand electrode
Migraine	9.5	Plate electrode on the forehead	Plate electrode in the neck
Tiredness	2.2	2 connected hand electrodes	2 connected foot electrodes
Muscle cramp	6.8	Supply with hand or foot electrodes, depending on the location of the affected muscles	

Myoma	2.5	Foot electrode on the myoma side or vaginal electrode	Foot electrode on the opposite side or place plate electrode into the small of the back
Neck stiffness	9.4	Plate electrodes as for circulatory problems or roll electrode for rolling the hand electrode myalgias	
Otoscle-rosis	9.2	Hand electrodes, possibly add another 3.3 Hz when combined with arte-riosclerosis, or active auditory canal electrode on the same side	
Pan-creatic disorder	4.0	Hand electrode	Hand electrode
Paresthe-sia in the hands	9.1	As for circulatory problems	
Pareses	9.4	Treat area of paresis with roll electrodes	Hand or foot electrode
Phlebitis	10.0	Place active electrode on the inflamed veins, inactive foot electrode as longitudinal supply or inactive electrode on the opposite side as cross-supply, or above the end of the phlebitis as diagonal supply.	
Insomnia	2.5	Place active electrode onto forehead and eyes, inactive plate electrodes into the neck Note To get contact with the eyes, place damp cotton wool on the eyes and then the moist electrode supra-orbital and on check bone. One may, however only apply aligned positive pulses (PP) to avoid flashing on the retina. Reduce down to at least LW 70	
Cold	2.9	Plate electrode on the side with the stronger complaints	Plate electrodes on the opposite neck side
Weak-ness in the knees	3.5	Attach foot electrodes or plate electrodes to both sides of knee for cross-supply	
Sinusitis/ paranasal sinusitis	2.5	Plate electrode on the affected head and maxillary sinus	Plate electrode in the neck

Tachycardia	1.2	Hand electrode in the left hand	Hand electrode in the right hand
Ulcus duodeni/ ventriculi	9.4	Hand electrode	Hand electrode
Circulatory disorders	9.4	For disorders in legs use both foot electrodes, for disorders in the arms use both hand electrodes or place one moist inactive plate electrode on the neck and take 2 coupled tube electrodes as active electrodes with special cable in both hands (three electrode treatment)	
Varices	9.4	Place plate electrode above the varicose veins	Foot electrode
Shaking	3.5	Hand electrode	Hand electrode

The beneficial Dr. Schüssler cell salts should be known to every therapist. To achieve the greatest possible anabolic effect, the knowledgeable therapist will use highly-effective natural remedies in combination for every treatment. For example, acupuncture, Baunscheidt's treatment of 1848, neural therapy[6] and the necessary homeopathic injection preparations can be combined quite well. From this aspect, this creates a multi-kybernetic overall healing effect with organ strengthening character. Focusing on today's diseases of civilisation characterises a good therapist. The identification and treatment of allergies which occur ever more frequently in children and adults is deemed a priority. Bladder and kidney diseases, pain in the joints, visual impairment and skin disorders speak for themselves. They should be attended to in the same way as ENT diseases, headaches, gastro-intestinal diseases and when a cancerous process already exists. In short, all necessary measures must be undertaken to put the body into an eutonic state so that it is able to create good, positive and healing oscillations which please the soul and mind with their frequencies. Nothing else will then stand in the way of a happy existence. One generally hears and reads little about a correct metabolic process. The now described processes, which concern the overall metabolism, are probably a welcome refresher of the material learnt during training for naturopaths and physicians. Each cell requires, amongst other things, proteins, fat and carbohydrates. Through certain processes these deliver energy which is essential for the body's functions and to retain vital functions. Creating body heat, growth and creating new tissue. The proteins are the most important part of protoplasm (the cell's living substance). It contains hydrogen, oxygen, sulphur and carbon. There are also proteins which contain other substances and phosphorus. The protein is essentially dependent on the amino acids, as they are the actual elements of the protein molecules. The protein molecule needs an alkaline amino group with carboxylic acid for its synthesis. Long chains are created by the amino acid molecules which, as the preliminary stage of proteins, are called polypeptides. When protein is broken down, it is done so by splitting the peptide combination into one of the amino acids. There is a series of amino acids which the body cannot form itself. Those added amino acids which have the greatest similarity with our body, respectively its tissue, have the greatest nutritional value. However, not only meat but also many types of vegetables are indispensable protein providers. It requires at least 8 amino acids to keep the body healthy. They are termed essential amino acids. Not only protoplasm, but also blood plasma, hormones and enzymes require the nitrogen in the amino acids.

By metabolism we generally understand all chemical reactions in the body's tissues. One could also look at the term of metabolism as food utilization. With metabolism we differentiate between catabolism and anabolism. Catabolism is the breakdown metabolism while anabolism represents the build-up metabolism.

Fats, as another important component of food, find special significance in the triglycerides (neutral fats). It must, however, also be said that the body needs cholesterol for its metabolism.

If there is insufficient cholesterol available, the body itself produced a certain amount. The body needs cholesterol to neutralise mycoses (fungal infections).

The molecules of the neutral fats are created from the combination of three fatty acid molecules and one glycerine molecule. Most fats are mixtures of two or more glycerides. Depending on how many hydrogen atoms exist, unsaturated and saturated fatty acids. The unsaturated fatty acids pass into those with less hydrogen, for example oleic acid. The saturated fatty acids include palmitic acid.

The third important factor in the compounds is the carbohydrates which consist of small molecules. They are combined of carbon and water. Important carbohydrates are monosaccharides and glucose. Glucose occurs in sweet fruits. When two monosaccharides are combined and a water molecule is eliminated, the result is cane sugar (sucrose) as a disaccharide. Starch is a polysaccharide which consists of many monosaccharides. Carbohydrates can be produced by the body itself from proteins and fats. Carbohydrates provide energy through oxidation (combination of a compound with oxygen). The carbohydrates are stored as supplies in the form of glycogen and can be converted to fat when required. In the case of fats, oxidation also releases energy and stores it as fat. However, the body can also convert fats to sugar.

Proteins can be converted to fat but also to sugar. They can also be used in synthesis. Here too proteins can be turned to energy via oxidation. There is a great difference between digestion and metabolism. Digestion means converting food into substances which are absorbed by the lymph system and the blood. Metabolism is the utilization of the digested food by the cell. A significant product of metabolism is the resultant carbon dioxide. Glucose, however, is a substance from carbohydrate digestion.

We are familiar with electrical, chemical, mechanical and thermal energy in the context of our body. Chemical energy is of great importance to our body as it is necessary for cell functions. It is created through the breakdown of carbohydrates, fats and proteins. It is either stored or used, depending on requirement. When muscles are used, we need chemical energy. The organism uses the major part of chemical energy as thermal energy and heat regulation via the skin, either as evaporation or perspiration regulation. The body produces a certain heat under variable conditions and this is then termed basal metabolic rate. A number of calories is generated in a certain period under determination of the percentile change of a standard value. An indication about the processes in the cells is thus given via chemical processes. The basal metabolic rate is different for every person. It is subject to various factors such as gender, thyroid hyperfunction or hypofunction or sleep. Approximately 70% of the body consists of water. It is distributed into cell fluid, the space between the cell, respectively tissue and the blood vessels. Excretion takes place via the kidneys, intestine, lung and skin. To keep the tissue fluids going, a person requires 2-2.5 litres of fluid per day. If too much water collects in the interstitium (between the cells) one speaks of an oedema. Toxins increase the permeability of the vessel wall. An oedema can also occur through the occlusion of a lymph vessel. Sometimes the hydrostatic pressure in the capillaries rises in the case of venous occlusion or cardiac insufficiency. The protein metabolism additionally regulates the hydrostatic pressure in the blood vessels. This depends on the production of the proteolytic enzymes in the pancreas. Acidic end products occur during cell metabolism. This results in an increase of the hydrogen ions in the body fluids. The pH value of 7 documents a neutral solution in the blood. The pH value of 7.35 − 7.45 is maintained by carbonic acid and hydrogen carbonate in a corresponding ratio. The body attempts to prevent changes to the blood pH with its blood buffers where sodium hydrogen carbonate is the most important buffer for an acid-base regulation. Phosphate, protein and carbonate buffers are further important pH value regulators. There is additional buffering via the kidneys and respiration. When carbon dioxide is breathed out, the acid concentration in the organism falls. A weak respiratory function results in an increase of the carbon dioxide concentration. Too heavy breathing (hyperventilation) withdraws too much carbon dioxide from the body, causing the pH value to rise strongly. We then speak of an alkalosis which itself causes damage when the pH value rises too high. This can lead to psychic disorders, oxygen deficiency and liver diseases or even be brought forward from there. Kidneys are involved in buffering through reabsorption of hydrogen carbonate. The pH value of urine is naturally somewhat acidic. However, to be able to excrete waste products and toxins from the body, urin should have a pH value of 6.8 to 7 between 3 p.m. and 3 a.m.

Of all the body systems, the nervous system is the most developed. It makes it possible for mankind to register and understand his environment. The interaction of the body systems is regulated by the nerves. Protoplasm has the property of nervous conduction within the nervous system. Impulses are created within the nerve fibres and these transmit at high speed along the nerve pathways to their destination. They transfer information, which is necessary for the regulation of body functions. Our nervous system harbours three different cell types.

The neurons as the main nerve cells, the so-called glia and the small, respectively microscopic glial cells. The glia are responsible for the connective tissue of the nervous system.

The micro glia have the ability of disposing decomposition products from the cells, which occur when cells decompose.

The neurons as the actual nerve cells contain three types of nervous conduction.

The feeding neurons conduct the stimuli formed by the protoplasm to the spinal cord or brain.

The motoric neurons conduct the stimuli away from the central nervous system. The switching neurons transfer impulses from the efferent neurons. They also conduct the impulses away from the afferent neurons.

The neuron as nerve cell with its cytoplasm consists of the cell body and one to several processes called dendrites. The longer processes are called axon or neurite. The dendrites conduct the stimuli to the inside of the nerve cell and the neurite conducts the stimuli away from the cell. If an impulse jumps from one neuron to another neuron, the touchpoint is called a synapse. It connects two nerve cells with each other. When this mechanism is disrupted, it results in states such as fear, depression and/or aggressiveness.

We distinguish three parts of the nervous system: spinal cord and brain constitute the central nervous system as well as the nervous system situated to the outside, which consists of cerebral and spinal nerves. The third part is the autonomous nervous system with its network of fibres and ganglia. It supplies the smooth muscles of the digestive tract and the cardiac vessel system. It also supplies the glands and is divided into the parasympathetic and sympathetic nervous system (vegetative system). The spinal nerves exit the spine as 31 nerve pairs. They supply the cervical, thoracic, lumbar and sacral segments. There is also a coccyx nerve. From the top down, the spinal nerves divide into eight cervical, twelve thoracic, five lumbar, five sacral nerves and one coccyx nerve.

The central nervous system supplies all regions of the organism except the internal organs, while the autonomous nervous system (vegetative system) regulates the unconscious body functions. This includes regulation of gland activity and cardiac function. By nature, the sympathetic and parasympathetic trunk should be in balance, effecting psychic wellbeing. They provide energy and mobilise, similar to the action of the hormones adrenalin and noradrenalin, the body for flight, defence and combat readiness. When the heart is just short of failure, the blood pressure is slightly raised but the vegetative system is nearly normal (which can be determined with a BFD all-round measurement according to Dr. Voll), the patient is in his last survival battle without him being aware of this at times. This has been observed quite often where an ECG, even under stress, always only ever means the energetic dissipation and gives no information about the cardiac muscle strength. To have healthy oscillations of its overall function act on the mind and soul in total, a major part of the body is the body's own defence system. The RES as reticuloendothelial system is a reticular (netlike) composition of defence cells especially in the area of the connective tissue. The inside of the blood and lymph vessels is lined with defence cells. These are cells which absorb non-physiological substances, bacteria and viruses. They are also able to produce antibodies if so required. These specific cells can also be found in the bone marrow, in the liver and in the lymphatic spleen as well as in lymph nodes. There are also cells which can pass through tissue to ingest foreign bodies. So-called haemocytoplasts are formed in the red bone marrow and these develop into erythrocytes. The leukocytes develop from the myeloplasts (bone marrow cells). The lymphocytes and histiocytes develop in the lymph nodes, which, once they have passed through tissue, seek out microorganisms and ingest these. In the liver and spleen reticulum cells eliminate and dissolve foreign bodies. They are also able to form plasma cells which produce certain defence bodies which can then, in turn, destroy foreign substances. The white blood count contains five different blood corpuscles all of which have a defence function. If cells are damaged, they give off mikrosin into their environment. Mikrosin raises the permeability of the capillaries. Blood protein can thus enter the inflamed tissue. The fibrin takes care of clotting and this provides a protective wall around the focus of inflammation. From this aspect, it is a protection against the spread of bacteria. Other defence bodies and mechanisms also play a part.

As already mentioned above, hormones and enzymes regulate all processes within the body where, however, organ strengthening and detoxification are in the foreground. Detox by means of strengthening the excretory organs and removal via the skin take priority. The hormonal system consists of hormone glands which give their hormones off straight into the blood. These are glands without excretory ducts. We differentiate between glands with excretory ducts which give off their fluids into a body cavity or into the external region of the organism.

The pituitary gland is divided into three sections. The front part (adenohypophysis) is superior and has an effect on the other hormonal glands. These are the thyroid gland, ovaries, testes, as well as adrenal glands and thymus gland. The pituitary gland also influences the gastro-intestinal tract. Certain hormones reach the bloodstream from there. The hormone excretion by the adenohypophysis is controlled by a feedback mechanism. By contrast, the posterior pituitary excretes the hormones oxytocin and vasopressin. These effect the contraction of the womb during the birthing procedure. Under the effect of the pituitary gland, the thyroid gland excretes growth hormones. The parathyroid gland as four small epithelial bodies on the back of the thyroid gland make up the so-called parathormone, which influences the calcium metabolism. A deficiency causes muscle cramps which can lead to death. The development of osteoporosis is also dependent on the parathyroid gland.

The adrenal glands as the most important hormonal glands are located on the kidneys. They produce around 29 corticoids (cortisone-like substances). They are indispensable when it comes to the production of antibodies and the metabolism of fats and carbohydrates. They build adrenalin in the adrenal medulla which has a similar effect as the sympathetic nerve. Noradrenalin from the adrenal glands is involved in the constriction of the vessels and therefore with a rise in blood pressure.

The pancreas is another hormonal gland with the islands of Langerhans and their insulin production, which channel the blood sugar into the cells. Insufficient insulin can lead to death or coma, however, it manifests first as diabetes mellitus. The ovaries are located in the female major pelvis. They give off the oestrogen and progesterone into the blood. They are necessary for menstruation and the functioning of the sexual organs. Menstrual disorders are usually due to a lack of oestrogen, as are underdeveloped breasts. If there is insufficient progesterone it also causes menstrual disorders and loss of the foetus in pregnant women. A regular hormone status is therefore necessary for women who are affected in this way. The male testes produce the male gametes and the testosterone.

The thymus gland is an important defence organ and lies behind the sternum. The epiphysis is located in the middle brain and it seems to have an influence on the sleeping rhythm.

Hormones are also produced in the digestive tract. The stomach lining produces only gastrin which is required for digestion. The gastrin also stimulates the pancreas. Cholecystokinin effects the contraction of the gall bladder muscles so that about 30 minutes after eating, bile flows into the small intestine. The hormone enterogastron, which is excreted by the duodenum, inhibits the excretion of gastric juices. The enzymes, which catalyse the metabolic processes in the body should find particular attention. The enzymes develop optimum effect when the blood is slightly base. The pancreas produces, for example, enzymes which, as specific proteins, are essential for fat, carbohydrate and protein breakdown. Enzymes also attack the sheath of tumour cells and dissolve these so that the tumour cell is identifiable for the body's own defence and can be eliminated only then. The enzyme mechanism also grabs the adhesion molecules which are on the tumour cell. These enable the tumour cell to cling to the vessel walls, a process which effects the creation of metastases. An enzyme deficiency can be prevented by taking corresponding substances. A high-dose enzyme therapy is recommended in the case of cancerous processes. No matter which reactions occur in the body, enzymes are always involved. As particularly effective proteins they accelerate all processes in the body. If the organism lacks certain enzymes it leads to serious dysfunctions. These develop into diseases and their course which could be prevented by the right substitution. Even in ancient times one knew how to make use of the enzyme effect when brewing beer or making cheese and wine. Enzymes not only accelerate the reactions in the body but they can also effect reactions. Proteins are split by proteases. The fats require their lipases and the carbohydrates are dependent on the activity of the amylases to be split up. The proteases for splitting protein are chymotrypsin, trypsin, bromelain, papain etc. The effect of the enzymes is based on compounds they engage in and change with the components but where they subsequently change again. The concentration of the hydrogen ions and the respective enzyme substrate influence the cleavage process. If the pH value falls into the acidic range the enzyme activity falls. Enzyme assays depend on how strong the enzyme activity is. Chymotrypsin is, similar to trypsin, a proteolytic (protein splitting) enzyme. It is found mainly in the duodenal juice. The stomach produces 1 g pepsinogen daily in its fundic glands. The hydrochloric acid of the stomach activates pepsinogen to pepsin. It participates in the digestive action in the stomach. So that the mucous lining of the stomach is not attacked, it is protected by inhibitors. The enzyme papain is won from the papaya fruit. Papain has an anti-inflammatory effect. Papaya is a valuable help in the case of worm infections.

The fat splitting lipases from tissues and the pancreas have a pH value of 90. They have the capacity of splitting fats into fatty acids.

Amylases can be found in fungi and the pancreas. They split glycogen and starch into maltose (malt sugar). If the pancreas produces insufficient enzymes they can be added successfully by simply taking them. This increases the enzyme content in the blood. A lack of pancreatic enzymes effects inadequate digestion of the ingested food. If there is a hypoacidity of the stomach, the therapist will administer a pepsin-hydrochloric acid preparation. The popular pancreas powder contains carbohydrate, fat and protein splitting enzymes. Sugar coated pills release their enzymes in the small intestine. They should be taken before meals as digestive enzyme. Meteorism (collection of gas) occurs in the intestinal region if there is a lack of digestive enzymes. One then speaks of a general digestive insufficiency with involvement of the liver and gall bladder. Preventive taking is advised when meals rich in protein and fats, as well as meals which are hard to digest, are on the menu.

People today reach a higher age than at the time of the turn of the century (around 1900). The causes lie in a better hygiene, more targeted combating of infectious diseases, and in particular a healthier, more broadly based nutrition rich in vital substances. Hunger and epidemics or plagues are nearly non-existent in the developed countries.

However, nearly every second person in the industrial states dies of arteriosclerosis. Enzymes, which have a fibrinolytic (dissolve fibrin) effect, reduce or prevent arteriosclerosis. In the case of a high-dose application the result is a microscopic decomposition of already existing, deposited fibrinolytic fibres and plaques of the intima (internal vascular membrane). These are not only cholesterol deposits but also protein residues which have a major contribution towards the formation of plaques. In addition to the cardiac overacidification, many a heart attack and/or stroke are due to a coronary sclerosis. Inflammations, which occur with almost all illnesses, play a large role in this. The inflammation usually represents the last defence in the subacute happenings of pathological processes before the chronic stage. And even then - in cases of exception -, inflammations occur in the chronic occurrences, which accompany the disease process in a somewhat changed form. An inflammation where the organism has to battle with an overload of the body with toxins, waste products and a flood of acid is particularly stubborn. Battling the inflammation with cortisone and salicylates can only ever be crowned by brief success. In addition, the damaging side effects affect the whole organism. If, however, one resorts to enzymes to get control of inflammatory processes, the body receives the non-toxic help which does no damage. Even in the case of a permanent therapy there are no undesirable side effects which would justify a short application. If the capillaries extend during the inflammatory process, fluid issues into the tissue and swellings occur which themselves cause additional complaints. A fibrin concentration at the site of an inflammation is necessary there for blot clotting. Toxic substances are enclosed when a clot forms. This puts a stop to further spread of the process. Fibrin is created when the preliminary stage of fibrin, the fibrinogen, comes into contact with damaged tissue. This already happens before the leukocytes appear at the "battle site". However, the fibrin is also responsible for circulatory disturbances in the region of inflammation. This then causes stasei, swellings and pain around the local inflammation. The plasmin as proteolytic enzyme attempts to dissolve the sluggish fluids. This process is supported by taking enzyme preparations. At the beginning of the inflammation, the building of fibrin is important to seal things off at the stated site, however, it should be dissolved again after new cells, respectively tissue have formed. This is possible by taking a higher dose of enzymes. If the generously produced fibrin is not dissolved quickly enough, pathological process will occur in the organism.

New research has shown that deposits in the vessels can be broken down microscopically through high doses of enzymes and excessive new production is prevented. This process is called physiological fibrinolysis. Enzymes are also required when thromboses have occurred in vessels. High-dose enzyme substitution with cancer has led to a better progress in many cases and should find more attention in oncology.

In 1938 Dr. Seeger[7] had already found out that a steady increase of toxins in the body leads to respiratory disorders of the cells. This means that less and less oxygen and vital nutrients reach the cells. The toxins and waste products produced during cell metabolism can no longer be eliminated. From the aspect of the physiological processes, the results are serious disorders which show up as illnesses. An unblocking of the respiration of the affected cell membranes with antiferment blocking injections becomes necessary. This way it is possible to re-instate the permeability of the cell boundary membrane. Oxygen and nutrients increasingly reach the cells, waste products and toxins are eliminated to relieve the cells. Many a cell can leave the fermentation metabolism and return to normal metabolism. The related symptoms can be reduced or even totally eliminated.

The mysterious entity of the Major Three

Every being is an existence. Every being lives through a body, a mind and a soul which in turn are an entity and which merge harmoniously in a constant correlation. If one part of this entity experiences a disorder, the total coherence of mind-body-soul gets out of balance. The healthy, vital harmony is disturbed.

To rephrase:

The harmonious triad of body-mind-soul receives nourishment from the surrounding, cosmic oscillations, divine energies which are in unison with it. If this harmonious triad then meets oscillations which cannot fit harmoniously into the own pattern of the mind or soul, or into the own body oscillations, the whole structure experiences disharmony. If the soul gets out of step as a result of unexpected strokes of fate, both the mind and body suffer. If thoughts are troubled by serious problems, this again impairs the body's wellbeing and the emotional balance. An ill body also deprives its soul and mind of the necessary strength.

The soul in the mysterious triad

In this entity of the major three, the soul probably represents the most sensitive, vulnerable part.

The beginning, new life, already takes up the mother's oscillations while still in the womb. The child's soul oscillates in unison with the mother's soul. Therefore, if the mother's soul is in a harmonious order, the child feels wanted, loved, accepted and secure. It will have a good and healthy development. However, what happens if the mother suffers emotional mood swings?

Perhaps the child is an "accident" and doesn't fit into the current life plans, there is controversy with the partner, the child's father leaves the mother, fears for the future make a presence, job loss, termination of the living quarters, the death of a close person. All these things and more first affect the mother's soul. It looses its harmonious order. The child's soul receives the inappropriate oscillations, and its wellbeing, the state of its soul is impaired. These impairments then disrupt the mother's metabolism, the immune system weakens, the organs loose their strength and can no longer supply the child adequately. Complications are the result and these can lead all the way to the death of the child. Of course it is not always possible to protect the soul and withdraw from everything that is negative. A good immune system which can handle stress, strong organs, good metabolism, a healthy acid-base household, however, can keep the physical effects of emotional imbalance within boundaries.

The soul needs a counterpart. The soul needs communication. The oscillations of two souls meet and form a whole. As already described above, the soul of the unborn child communicates with the mother's soul.
The souls of small children communicate with the oscillations of their parents, siblings, friends and the persons around them. If the child grows up in a harmonious family environment, the oscillations of the individual family members are in unison. The child's physical, mental and emotional strength grows! It can develop harmoniously.
A harmonious whole in the family means that conflicts must happen occasionally. Conflicts are part of life and are dealt with on the mental level. The soul doesn't have to suffer through the conflict. The opposite is true. The soul is strengthened. It also learns to ward off, learns to compensate stress. The good measure of harmony and sense of conflict strengthen the energetic oscillations of each soul, especially in the harmonious family union. It is the parent's duty to develop a sensible "dispute culture". In an intact, harmonious rela-

tionship emotional blows below the belt should never be included when engaging in a conflict

Children can immediately feel the difference between verbal, emotional injuries or a factual, mental discussion.

If the child, however, is surrounded by a climate which is characterised by disharmonies, it weakens the filial soul. It withers. Children immediately detect even the smallest changes in mood without knowing the reason. Their soul is still pure, unspent and therefore very receptive for changes in oscillations. But it can also be hurt very quickly. It can loose its order very quickly. This then influences the metabolism. The immune system and the organs become weaker, the intoxication in the body rises. Aggressiveness, hyperactivity, lethargy, exhaustion, sleep disorders, feelings of fear, allergies and chronic disorders are the result. The child's soul cries out for harmony, cryies for help to have order reinstated.

"She's a good soul!" "He's a soul of a person!" Many of these statements have long been a part of our language. What they mean is clear to everyone. One person stands in for the other, helps his counterpart, supports him, listens, and is simply there for the other. One soul is there for the other. Takes care of it, helps to regain order. It helps it to find its oscillations again.

While doing this, the helping soul can also grow. It can pass its positive oscillations on.

Souls need a counterpart. Souls need communication. Otherwise they wither. Otherwise they grow lonely and become ill.

"It is not good that the man should be alone!" This quote from the Bible contains a high degree of truth. In today's age where independence, freedom and self- fulfilment take top priority we are hardly dependent on anyone else anymore. Each person can manage on his or her own. But how does a soul feel with all of this?

The time will come when the soul feels the loneliness. Its energy of being there for others, but also to absorb other energies and strengthen itself from these, dwindles.

The person feels depressive, listless, lacks drive, and is dissatisfied, sullen, and lonely. He looses his view of life. He looses his sense of life. He then often reacts in a manner incomprehensible to others. His soul cries out for a YOU!

The stress through lack of the counterpart leads to disturbances of the metabolism, impairments in the body's organism. If there is, in addition, a high total toxic stress of the organ system, it inevitably comes to impairments in the cerebral nerve cells. The result is often that not enough neurotransmitters (carrier substances) are developed. The nerve impulses at the synapse (point where the nerve cells touch) cannot jump adequately from one cell to the other. Depending on predisposition, this leads to depression, states of fear or also aggressive behaviour.

The dimension of all being is the invisible divine power which penetrates everything. Depending on how the fine oscillations between two persons are felt, there is a chance of getting onto the track of the secret of creation. Every person is different and also differentiates himself through his charisma which comes from inside. It is particularly important to respect the other person's personality and not only to use him. According to the divine laws, the correlation of the inner oscillations would automatically change in this case and the deeper bonds would dissolve. The result would be an end to the still existing mysterious sense of togetherness. This then peaks in the fact that the one no longer understands the other. Perhaps this partial aspect is also a part of the deeper secrets of life, which no one has really been successfully in tracking down finally. It seems that the inexhaustible, unlimited and infinite of another dimension adhere to the divine secret. If the oscillations of one partner in a relationship change towards the other partner in a negative direction, the partners distance themselves from each other.

There are people with special talents. Close persons find it phenomenal to puzzling. What is the reason why people keep being born who are especially talented? Could it not actually be that these talents are experiences from an earlier life? We are all tied into many different relationships. The relationship of all living beings to the moon also represents a special relationship. The hygroscopic effect of the moon is reflected, amongst other things, in the example of the low and high tides of the oceans. The different phases of the moon also have an influence on all living beings. Blood pressure rises at full moon, the heart rate is raised and the hormone production is increased. When the moon wanes, the body, soul and mind are unburdened.

The new moon between the waning and waxing moon promotes energy, vitality and concentration. Body and soul are relaxed best, for example, during meditation. The waxing moon promotes optimism and energy. Eroticism and passion are in a favourable stage, as the body produces more happiness hormones and the soul oscillates in harmony.

Bibliography

Voll, R. "Topographische Messpunkte nach Dr.Voll", medizinisch literarische Verlagsgesellschaft Uelzen, 1977.

Pschyrembel, W. "Klinisches Wörterbuch", Verlag de Gruyter, Berlin, Germany, 1975.

Seeger, Dr. "Gibt es eine Präkanzerose ?"

Neunhoeffer, Prof. Dr. med. F., "Möglichkeiten und Aussagekraft biochemisch bedingter Laboratoriumsteste für Krebs, Krebsgeschehen", 8/1976H5, S.110.

Neunhoeffer, Prof. Dr. med. F., "Die biochemischen Abweichungen der entarteten Zelle und die Konsequenzen für Krebsteste und Krebstherapie" Band 12, Verlag für Medizin, Dr. Ewald Fischer GmbH, Heidelberg, Germany, 1978.

Gutschmidt, Dr. J., "Die Carcinochromreaktion".

Scheller, E.F. "Hämatologische Krebsfrühdiagnostik".

"Baunscheidt", Ariston-Verlag (Hrsg.) Geneva, Switzerland, 1976.

Schroedter, Sonderdruck aus "Krebsgeschehen und Praxis der Onkologie", Hrsg. H. Denk, K. Karrer, G. Salzer, Vienna, Austria.

Seeger, Dr. P.G., "Präkanzerose und ist diese aufspürbar", Erfahrungsh.K. 28, 1979 K.4, S. 244.

Das Lymphsystem und das Retikuloendothelial-System, Verlag Chemie GmbH, 6940 Weinheim, Germany, 1976.

List of sources

Das Endokrinsystem, Verlag Chemie GmbH Weinheim, Bergstraße, Germany,1971.

Arterienverkalkung Dr. med. Kurt Pollack, Paracelsusverlag Stuttgart, 3rd edition, 1971.

Culclasure, David. Das Ernährungs- und Stoffwechselsystem, Verlag Chemie GmbH Weinheim, Bergstraße, Germany,1971.

Culclasure, David. Das Nervensystem, Verlag Chemie GmbH Weinheim, Bergstraße, Germany, 1976.

Rausberger, Karl und Wolf, Max. Enzymtherapie, Wilhelm Maudrich Verlag, Vienna, Austria, 1970.

Murphy, Joseph Dr., Die Macht Ihres Unterbewusstseins, Aristonverlag, Geneva, Switzerland, 1962.

Rietig, Wolfgang, "Phänomen" Plötzlicher Kindstod – endlich erkannt, BOD-Verlag, Norderstedt, Germany, 2007.

Rietig, Wolfgang, Gesund oder Erschöpft ? Ganzheitstherapie/Naturheilkunde Schmerz-Herz-Kreislauf-Krebs", BOD-Verlag, Norderstedt, Germany,2008.
("Healthy or exhausted? **Holistic therapy/Naturopathy Pain-Heart-Circulation-Cancer").**

Rietig, Wolfgang, "Länger aktiv leben! Entsäuern – Entschlacken – Entgiften. Krebserkrankung – Krebsprophylaxe", BOD-Verlag, Norderstedt, Germany, 2009.

(Living a longer active life! Deacidifying-Cleansing-Detoxing. Cancer-Cancer prophylaxis").

Endnotes

1   Pherecydes of Syros.
2   Comp. Dr. Joseph Murphy.
3   Comp. Dr. Joseph Murphy.
4   According to Baunscheidt 1848, elimination method via the skin.
5   Dr. Voll operated and further developed EAP (electro-acupuncture) and BFD.
6   Developed by the physicians Walter and Ferdinand Huneke (Therapy via the nervous system).
7   Dr. Seeger, cancer researcher.